THE POWER OF FOOD

Harnessing Nutrition For Diabetes Control

RUTH PETERS

COPYRIGHT

TABLE OF CONTENT

INTRODUCTION

Welcome to this amazing journey of managing diabetes with diet. The goal of this book is to provide people with diabetes with the knowledge and tools they need to take charge of their health through proper nutrition and a well-balanced diet. You can successfully manage your diabetes and lead a full and healthy life by making informed food choices, comprehending how various nutrients affect blood sugar levels, and creating a customized meal plan.

Although managing diabetes can be difficult, it need not be overwhelming. With the appropriate information and resources, you can adopt lifestyle changes that will result in better blood sugar regulation, more energy, and a lower chance of problems. This book will work as your all-inclusive guide, giving you insightful information, useful advice, and evidence-based approaches to managing diabetes with nutrition.

We will establish the groundwork in the first chapter by learning everything there is to know about diabetes. We'll look at the many forms of diabetes, their origins and risk factors, potential complications that could develop if diabetes is not effectively controlled, and so on. This information will give the nutritional solutions described throughout the book a strong basis.

The crucial role that diet plays in the management of diabetes is covered in detail also. You'll learn how various foods affect blood sugar levels, about glycemic load and index, and about the role that macronutrients (carbohydrates, proteins, and fats) and micronutrients play in preserving good health.

With this information in hand, the next chapter walks you through the process of developing a meal plan that is suitable for people with diabetes. We will go over goal-setting, portion control, and creating a balanced meal. You will also discover useful methods for organizing your meals and how to work in healthy snacks into your daily schedule.

Carbohydrates, proteins, and lipids are topics equally discussed. You will learn more about carbs and their effect on blood sugar regulation, as well as the necessity of proteins and fats in a diabetes diet will next be discussed, along with the optimum sources and amounts to consume in order to maintain general health and properly control blood sugar levels.

We shall delve into the foods to emphasize and the foods to limit or avoid in a diabetes diet, you will learn about the strength of non-starchy vegetables, lean meats, healthy fats, and whole grains and fiber. In order to promote the best possible management of your diabetes, we will also talk about the necessity of reducing or eliminating sugars, processed foods, high-sodium meals, and harmful fats from your diet.

As you read this book, we'll provide you with useful tips, healthy recipes for your breakfast, lunch, dinner, snacks and dessert, as well as healthy homemade drinks for your maximum enjoyment. You may improve your overall quality of life, control your blood sugar levels more effectively, lower your risk of problems, and take charge of your nutrition.

Let's now get out on this adventure together and learn how diet-based diabetic management may change lives.

CHAPTER 1

AN OVERVIEW OF DIABETES

Millions of individuals throughout the world suffer with diabetes, a complicated and chronic metabolic illness. It is defined by the body's inability to control blood sugar levels adequately, resulting in chronic hyperglycemia. The inability of the pancreas to adequately generate or use the hormone insulin, which helps control blood glucose levels, is the cause of this illness. Diabetes has serious health concerns and needs to be managed for the rest of one's life to prevent complications and preserve quality of life. We will give a general summary of diabetes, covering its kinds, causes, symptoms, and probable side effects.

Diabetes comes in a variety of forms, each with unique symptoms and causes. The most typical varieties include:

1. Type 1 Diabetes: Type 1 diabetes, sometimes referred to as juvenile diabetes or insulin-dependent diabetes, typically manifests during childhood or adolescence. It happens when the body's immune system unintentionally targets and kills the pancreatic cells that make insulin. Type 1 diabetics must administer insulin intravenously or employ an insulin pump to control their blood sugar levels.

2. Type 2 Diabetes: Type 2 diabetes, which accounts for the majority of diabetes occurrences worldwide, is the most common type. Insulin resistance, which occurs when the body's cells grow resistant to the actions of insulin and raise blood sugar levels, is what distinguishes it. Obesity, sedentary habits, poor diet, and genetic predisposition are all known risk factors for type 2 diabetes. At first, oral medications and lifestyle changes may be advised, but some people may eventually need insulin therapy.

3. Gestational Diabetes: About 7% of pregnant women experience gestational diabetes, which manifests during pregnancy. It happens when the body's capacity to adequately utilise insulin is compromised by hormonal changes. Although postpartum gestational diabetes normally goes away, affected women are more likely to acquire type 2 diabetes in the future.

Depending on the type, diabetes can have a variety of distinct causes. The major cause of type 1 diabetes is thought to be an autoimmune reaction that is brought on by both genetic and environmental causes. Poor food decisions, inactivity, and obesity are all lifestyle variables that are significantly linked to type 2 diabetes. However, because those who have a family history of type 2 diabetes are more at risk, genetic factors also play an important role. Ageing, ethnicity (such as being of African, Hispanic, or Asian heritage), and a history of gestational diabetes are additional risk factors for type 2 diabetes.

Depending on the type and severity of the disease, diabetes symptoms might change. Typical warning signs and symptoms include:

1. Constant thirst and urinating a lot

2. Unaccounted-for weight loss

3. Weakness and exhaustion

4. Vision haziness

5. Slow-healing injuries and illnesses

6. Numbness or tingling in the hands or feet

7. Repeated infections, particularly those of the urinary tract

It is crucial to remember that some people with type 2 diabetes may not exhibit obvious symptoms at first, which might result in instances going untreated.

Diabetes that is not under control might have serious side effects on the body's organ systems. Chronic hyperglycemia can harm blood vessels, resulting in cardiovascular issues like peripheral artery disease, heart disease, and stroke. Diabetic nephropathy, diabetic neuropathy, and diabetic retinopathy are additional conditions that are much more common in people with diabetes. Diabetes that is not well controlled can also weaken the immune system, increasing the risk of infection and delaying the healing of wounds. Diabetes also ups the chance of foot ulcers and amputations.

Diabetes is a common and difficult condition that needs ongoing management and care. Recognizing the many kinds, diabetes patients must be aware of the disease's causes, symptoms, and potential complications. Effective diabetes care requires early diagnosis, lifestyle changes (such as a healthy diet and frequent exercise), adequate medication adherence, and regular blood sugar monitoring. People with diabetes can reduce complications, improve their quality of life, and live long, healthy lives by taking a proactive approach to their care.

BLOOD SUGAR MONITORING

Monitoring blood sugar is essential to managing diabetes effectively. Maintaining ideal blood sugar levels is crucial for people with diabetes in order to avoid problems, improve general health, and enhance quality of life. Individuals can make educated decisions regarding their nutrition, exercise, and medication management with regular monitoring. The significance of blood sugar monitoring, various monitoring techniques, goal ranges, and the advantages it offers people with diabetes will all be covered in this section.

Monitoring blood sugar levels helps people understand the effects of numerous stimuli on their blood sugar levels and offers insightful information about how the body is metabolizing glucose. Regular blood sugar monitoring allows people to spot patterns, modify their diabetes management strategy as needed, and evaluate the success of both lifestyle changes and medication.

There are various monitoring techniques, like;

Self-Monitoring of Blood Glucose (SMBG): SMBG entails measuring blood sugar levels at home with a glucometer. A little blood sample is normally taken via finger prick, and the glucometer then analyzes it. This technique can be used several times each day and provides quick benefits. People are given the ability to make decisions about their food, exercise, and insulin dosage in real-time thanks to SMBG.

 Continuous Glucose Monitoring (CGM): CGM entails the use of a tiny sensor worn beneath the skin to continually track the amount of glucose present in the interstitial fluid. A receiver or smartphone app receives the data from the sensor, which provides real-time glucose levels and trends. In addition to providing a thorough perspective of daily glucose changes, including nighttime readings, CGM also enables users to spot patterns and trends that may go missed with SMBG alone.

Target blood sugar levels might vary depending on a person's age, type of diabetes, general health, and specific treatment objectives. The American Diabetes Association (ADA) generally suggests the pursuing target ranges:

1. Fasting Blood Sugar (4.4–7.2 mmol/L): 80–130 mg/dL before meals

2. After meals, postprandial blood sugar levels were 180 mg/dL (10.0 mmol/L).

Individual targets may differ, and healthcare professionals collaborate closely with patients to develop customised ranges tailored to their unique requirements.

There are numerous benefits associated with blood sugar monitoring, let's discuss a few of them

Optimal Diabetes treatment: People can fine-tune their diabetes treatment with the help of blood sugar monitoring. People can maintain blood sugar levels within goal limits by measuring their glucose levels on a regular basis and making prompt adjustments to their food, exercise, and medication regimens.

2. Prompt identification of bouts of hyperglycemia (high blood sugar) and hypoglycemia (low blood sugar) is made possible by regularly checking blood sugar levels. This enables people to act appropriately, such as modifying their insulin dosage, taking carbohydrates to boost blood sugar, or contacting a doctor as needed.

3. Appreciating the Effect of Food and Exercise: Monitoring blood sugar offers specific information on how various diets and physical activities affect glucose levels. Individuals can decide which choices result in optimal blood sugar control and make knowledgeable judgments about their daily routines by monitoring before and after meals or activity.

4. Personalized Diabetes Management: Monitoring blood sugar data enables fruitful conversations with healthcare professionals. It offers a thorough picture of a person's diabetes management, leading changes to medication, lifestyle advice, and goal-setting for the best possible diabetes care.

Monitoring blood sugar levels is an essential part of managing diabetes. By routinely checking blood sugar levels, people with diabetes can better understand their status, take control of their diet, exercise routine, and medication regimen, and manage their diabetes. Whether

on one's own monitoring of blood glucose, also known as continuous glucose monitoring, is a technique that enables people to take control of their health, optimize blood sugar levels, and lower their chance of developing diabetes-related illnesses. Individuals can actively control their diabetes and enhance their general well-being by prioritizing blood sugar monitoring.

CHAPTER 2

THE ROLE OF DIET IN DIABETES

One cannot overestimate the importance of nutrition in controlling blood sugar levels. Understanding how different foods affect blood glucose is crucial for people with diabetes to maintain good health and properly manage their condition. People can improve their blood sugar control, lower their risk of problems, and improve their general health by making educated food decisions. This section will examine the complex relationship between nutrition and blood sugar levels by looking at how proteins, carbs, and fats affect the control of glucose.

Blood sugar levels are most significantly influenced by carbohydrates. They decompose into glucose when ingested, raising blood sugar levels. But not every type of carbohydrate is the same. It is essential to comprehend the ideas of glycemic load (GL) and glycemic index (GI).

GLYCEMIC INDEX AND GLYCEMIC LOAD

The terms glycemic index (GI) and glycemic load (GL) are crucial in the context of nutrition and blood sugar control. These resources aid people in understanding how various meals affect blood sugar levels and assist them in making wise dietary decisions. Understanding the differences between glycemic load and glycemic index will help people better control their blood sugar, improve their general health, and lower their risk of problems. The definitions of GI and GL, their importance, and how they might be utilized to assist ideal blood sugar regulation will all be covered in this section

The glycemic index gauges how quickly a food's carbohydrates elevate blood sugar levels when compared to a reference food, often white bread or pure glucose. On a scale from 0 to 100, a number is given to each food. Blood sugar increases more slowly and gradually in response to foods with low GIs (below 55) than it does in response to high GIs (above 70). Most vegetables, whole grains, legumes, and fruits are examples of low GI foods that are digested and absorbed more slowly, resulting in a more stable blood sugar response. Processed grains, sweet snacks, and some fruits are examples of high GI foods that hasten the rise in blood sugar levels.

Glycemic load considers both the quality and quantity of carbs in a portion of food, whereas GI just considers the rate of carbohydrate absorption. Instead than focusing only on how quickly carbohydrates raise blood sugar, it takes into account the total amount of carbohydrates consumed.

Calculating GL involves calculating a food's GI by the quantity of carbs in a serving and dividing the result by 100. A high GL is usually 20 or above, whereas a low GL is frequently 10 or below. This measurement provides a more realistic picture of how a food will generally affect blood sugar levels.

In order to effectively control blood sugar levels, it can be helpful to understand the GI and GL of foods. They can be used as follows:

Picking Low GI Foods: Low GI foods are preferred since they have a milder effect on blood sugar levels. These include most fruits, whole grains (such as oats and quinoa), legumes, and non-starchy vegetables. These foods can help you maintain better blood sugar management by being included in your meals and snacks.

Pairing Carbohydrates with Protein and Healthy Fats: High GI meals can help slow down digestion and lower the total GI of a meal when they are combined with protein and healthy fats. An avocado or nut addition to a high GI fruit, for instance, can lessen the blood sugar surge.

Balancing Glycemic Load: It's crucial for blood sugar control to keep track of the GL of meals and snacks. People can attain improved blood sugar balance throughout the day by including a range of low and moderate GL foods and being aware of portion amounts.

Individual Considerations: It's crucial to remember that GI and GL levels might differ from person to person, and factors like general eating habits, medication use, and one's own health should also be taken into account. A certified dietitian or other healthcare expert can offer specific advice.

Understanding how various foods affect blood sugar levels can be done with the use of the glycemic index and glycemic load. People can improve blood sugar control and advance general health by including low GI and moderate GL foods in their meals, balancing carbohydrates with protein and fat, and paying attention to portion sizes. These ideas enable people to choose healthy diets, lower their risk of problems, and adopt a balanced approach to sugar control. Remember, creating a sustainable and individualized approach to nutrition that fits your specific needs and goals is more important than simply focusing on the numbers.

Although proteins and fats also contribute to the regulation of blood sugar, carbs have the biggest effect on blood sugar. Although they have little impact on blood sugar levels, proteins can help keep them stable when combined with carbohydrates. They lessen the speed at which carbs are broken down and absorbed, reducing sudden rises in blood sugar.

Blood sugar levels are not significantly influenced by lipids, even good fats such those found in avocados, almonds, and olive oil. However, they aid in general satiety and can slow down digestion, which results in more stable blood sugar levels. The effects of protein and fats in managing diabetes will be discussed in details later.

Several other elements outside macronutrients might affect blood sugar levels, elements like;

1. Fiber: Fiber, especially the soluble fiber present in whole grains, fruits, and vegetables, can slow down the digestion and absorption of carbohydrates, assisting in the maintenance of stable blood sugar levels.

2. Timing and Frequency of Meals: Eating smaller meals and snacks more frequently throughout the day can reduce the risk of significant blood sugar swings. Better glucose management may be supported by regular eating habits.

3. Alcohol: Drinking alcohol may interfere with the body's ability to control blood sugar, resulting in hypoglycemia or hyperglycemia. For people with diabetes, moderation and monitoring are crucial.

4. Hydration: Adequate hydration is crucial for the best blood sugar regulation. It's important to drink enough water throughout the day because dehydration might impact blood sugar levels.

For people with diabetes, maintaining blood sugar levels largely depends on diet. Making informed dietary decisions and achieving better blood sugar control require an understanding of how various foods affect the regulation of glucose. Individuals can improve their diet to support stable blood sugar levels by concentrating on balanced carbohydrate consumption, including proteins and healthy fats, and taking other aspects into account such as fiber, meal timing, and hydration.

Personalized meal plans should be created in close collaboration with healthcare professionals, such as registered dietitians or diabetes educators. With the right nutritional management, people can lead healthy, satisfying lives while successfully controlling their blood sugar levels and lowering their risk of developing diabetes-related problems.

MANAGING DIABETES WITH DIET

The management of diabetes heavily relies on diet. Making wise food decisions is crucial for people with this chronic illness in order to achieve optimal blood sugar control, avoid complications, and enhance overall health and well-being. People can take control of their health and start down the path to better diabetes management by knowing how various diet-related factors affect it. We will be discussing the significant impact of nutrition on diabetes management along with the need of a balanced and customized strategy, the role of macronutrients, portion control, and meal time.

Macronutrients

Carbohydrates: The greatest influence on blood sugar levels comes from carbohydrates. During digestion, they are converted into glucose, raising blood sugar levels. It's crucial to choose the correct kinds of carbohydrates and to watch your portion proportions. It can be beneficial to place an emphasis on complex carbs that have a low glycemic index, such as whole grains, legumes, and non-starchy vegetables.

Proteins: Lean meats, chicken, fish, tofu, and legumes are examples of foods high in protein that have little impact on blood sugar levels. They can support fullness, slow down the digestion of carbohydrates, and add to a balanced diet plan. Getting enough protein at meals and snacks helps with overall blood sugar control.

Fats: Consuming healthy fats, such those in avocados, nuts, seeds, and olive oil, is crucial for controlling diabetes. They promote heart health, assist control blood sugar levels, and promote satiety. However, because fat has a high calorie density, it is important to limit your intake.

Controlling Portion Size

Controlling portions is essential for managing diabetes. Eating in moderation aids in controlling blood sugar, preserving a healthy weight, and avoiding overeating. It is crucial to understand the recommended serving sizes for various food groups and to engage in mindful eating. Achieving portion control and boosting overall diabetes management can be facilitated by measuring food, utilizing smaller plates, and being conscious of hunger and fullness cues.

Timing and distribution of meals

For the control of diabetes, consistency in meal distribution and time is essential. Evenly spaced meals and snacks throughout the day aid in blood sugar stabilization, reduce significant swings, and maximize insulin absorption. Better blood sugar regulation can be facilitated by following a regular meal schedule and avoiding extended fasting.

Personalized Care and a Balanced Approach

Recognizing that diabetes management is extremely customized is vital. One person's ideal diet might not be suitable for another. Working closely with medical experts, such as certified diabetes educators or registered dietitians, can offer individualized advice and support. When planning a diet, a balanced approach takes into account cultural norms, personal preferences, and lifestyle concerns in order to achieve the best blood sugar control and general wellbeing.

While macronutrients are important, other elements also play a role in effective diabetes management;

 Dietary fiber, which may be found in fruits, vegetables, whole grains, and legumes, can help with blood sugar regulation, satiety, and digestive health. Keeping hydrated is crucial for managing diabetes.

Maintaining sufficient hydration and avoiding sugary beverages might help reduce unneeded blood sugar rises.

Consistent blood sugar monitoring, self-evaluation, and tracking of dietary decisions enable people to comprehend how their diet influences their control of diabetes. Meal plans can be modified using this information to encourage continued progress.

The management of diabetes heavily relies on diet. By being aware of how macronutrients affect health. People can improve blood sugar control, avoid problems, and enhance overall health by following a balanced and personalized approach, exercising portion control, emphasizing meal scheduling, and maintaining these healthy lifestyle habits. Taking control of diabetes management and leading a happy, healthy life are made possible by adopting a balanced diet and working with healthcare professionals. Always keep in mind that even modest adjustments can have a big impact, and that improving your diet will help you better manage your diabetes.

For a number of reasons, diet is important in the control of diabetes. Here are some crucial ideas emphasizing the role of diet in successfully managing diabetes:

Blood Sugar Control: Blood sugar levels are strongly impacted by diet. People can manage the quantity of glucose that enters their system and improve blood sugar control by eating the right meals and eating in moderation. Maintaining target blood sugar levels consistently lowers the likelihood of developing diabetes-related problems.

Weight management: A balanced diet helps a person reach and keep a healthy weight. A risk factor for type 2 diabetes, excess body weight might make blood sugar regulation more difficult. Individuals can limit their portion sizes, improve their insulin sensitivity, and manage their weight by including nutrient-dense foods into their diets.

Insulin Utilization: Diet affects how much insulin is used by the body and how it reacts to insulin. Certain meals, including carbs, directly affect how much insulin is needed. People can maximize insulin usage and lessen the need for medication modifications by picking the right carbohydrates, distributing them evenly throughout the day, and mixing them with proteins and healthy fats.

Complications can be prevented or managed with proper diet, which is important for diabetes-related complications. Dietary control of blood sugar levels can lower the risk of complications like heart disease, renal illness, nerve damage, and eye issues. An anti-inflammatory, antioxidant, and nutrient-rich diet can promote general health and lessen the effects of problems from diabetes.

Energy and Well-Being: A healthy diet offers the nutrients and energy required for overall wellbeing. The care of diabetes can be physically and emotionally taxing, but it is also important to maintain energy levels, mental clarity, and general quality of life through healthy nutrition. People can preserve their vitality, resiliency, and positive perspective by fueling their bodies with good foods.

In conclusion, eating is an essential component of managing diabetes since it affects weight management, the use of insulin, the reduction of complications, general wellbeing, and personal empowerment. People can improve their diabetes control, lower their risk of complications, and live a fuller, happier life with diabetes by adopting a healthy and balanced diet.

23

CHAPTER 3

CREATING DIABETES FRIENDLY MEAL PLAN

Setting goals for your food plan when controlling diabetes is a potent tactic that can enhance your general health and wellbeing. You can improve blood sugar control, alter your eating habits, and lower your risk of problems by setting specific, attainable goals. In this section, we'll discuss the significance of goal-setting for a diabetic meal plan and offer helpful advice to make and meet your nutritional objectives.

Setting goals provides you a sense of empowerment and motivation as you take charge of your diabetes management. It inspires you to make healthy changes to your eating habits and gives you the power to actively engage in your own health journey.

Goals also help you prioritize the improvements you want to accomplish by giving you clarity and direction. They act as a guide for your dietary decisions, ensuring that you stay on course and consistently move in the direction of greater health. Setting goals enables you to monitor your development over time. By establishing clear, quantifiable objectives, you can track your progress and mark significant turning points.

Here are some tips to help you in setting goals for diabetic friendly meals

Speak with a Healthcare Professional: Start by speaking with a certified diabetic educator or registered dietitian. They may offer you individualized advice, evaluate your unique needs, and assist you in creating goals that fit your lifestyle and tastes.

Be Specific and Realistic: Establish needs-based goals that are precise, measurable, and specific. Instead of aiming for general improvements like "eating healthier," for instance, focus on particular ones like "adding more vegetables to your meals" or "drinking less sugary beverages."

Gradual Changes: Concentrate on altering your dietary habits gradually. Instead of starting from scratch with your nutrition, set small, manageable goals and work your way up. This strategy helps you maintain long-term adjustments and improves your chances of success.

Make Portion Control a Top Priority: Portion control is essential for controlling blood sugar levels. Establish targets for portion control, such as using smaller plates, weighing food, or paying attention to serving sizes when dining out.

Place an emphasis on Balanced Nutrition: Strive to create a meal plan that is both nutritious and varied. Make it a point to include lean proteins, whole grains, fruits, vegetables, healthy fats, and all other dietary categories in your meals.

Pay attention to your carbohydrate consumption because it has a big impact on your blood sugar levels. Set objectives to select complex carbs with a low glycemic index, such as whole grains, legumes, and non-starchy vegetables, as your preferred source of fuel.

Setting goals to plan and prepare your meals in advance is another step. This supports maintaining consistency with your meal plan, avoiding impulsive eating, and making healthier decisions.

Regular Monitoring: Include objectives for routine blood sugar checking. This enables you to comprehend how your dietary decisions affect your blood sugar levels and adjust accordingly.

Recognize Progress: Honor your victories along the way. Recognize the tiny measures you take to achieve your objectives since they are important to your total achievement. Give yourself rewards that don't involve food and are related to your hobbies and interests.

Setting goals for your diabetes meal plan is an effective technique that gives you the power to take charge of your health and modify the way you eat. Setting clear, attainable, and measurable goals will help you concentrate your efforts, track your development, and achieve the best possible blood sugar control. Always place a priority on a healthy diet, and recognize your accomplishments as you go. You may set goals with a proactive mindset if you have a clear vision.

PORTION CONTROL

Portion control has become more crucial for keeping a healthy diet and controlling weight in today's environment of plentiful food options and bigger servings. Portion control is the conscious regulation of the amount of food eaten during a meal or snack. People can create a balanced eating pattern, improve general health, and avoid overeating by being aware of the advantages of portion management and putting them into practice. The importance of portion control, its advantages, and practical advice to help you implement it into your daily routine are all covered in this section.

Portion control is essential for calorie management. Overeating calories can result in weight gain, which increases the chance of developing a number of diseases like diabetes, heart disease, and obesity. People can achieve a calorie balance or deficit that supports weight management and a healthy body composition by using portion control techniques.

Also, Portion control is essential for persons who have diabetes or who want to keep their blood sugar levels stable. For efficient blood glucose management, the amount of carbohydrates ingested at each meal and snack must be balanced. People can better control their blood sugar and enhance their diabetes management by watching meal sizes and selecting the right carbohydrate sources.

 Portion management equally promotes a balanced diet that includes all the necessary nutrients. People can make sure they consume the right amount of protein, good fats, carbohydrates, vitamins, and minerals by managing their portion sizes. This balanced approach lowers the danger of vitamin deficiencies, maintains optimal bodily processes, and improves overall health.

Practicing and adopting portion control into your daily routine could be so easy, check out these easy tips

•Use Visual References: Get to know visual clues to gauge the proper portion sizes. For instance, a meal of carbs (like rice or pasta) should fit in the palm of your hand, a serving of fats (like oil or butter) should be the size of your thumb, and a serving of protein (like chicken or fish) should be around the size of a deck of cards.

•Read food labels and pay close attention to serving quantities. You can use this information to compare the recommended portion size to how much you really eat. Beware of packages that include numerous servings.

•Use Smaller Plates and Bowls: When serving meals, choose smaller plates and bowls. Your brain may be fooled into believing that a smaller portion will satisfy you by giving the impression that the plate is full.

• Measure and Weigh: To precisely measure servings, use measuring cups, spoons, and kitchen scales. This method gives a precise comprehension of the amount of food consumed and aids in gradually improving one's awareness of portion proportions.

•Prepare Meals Ahead of Time: Prepare meals and snacks ahead of time while taking into account portion sizes. This lessens the urge to overeat by enabling better control over the ingredients and portion amounts.

•Mindful Eating - Pay attention to your hunger and fullness signs while eating mindfully. Eat mindfully and deliberately, enjoying each meal, and stop when you are comfortably full rather than overstuffed.

•Seek Support: Tell loved ones or friends who can hold you accountable about your portion control goals. To create a customized portion control strategy, think about joining a support group or getting advice from a qualified dietitian or healthcare expert.

Portion control is an effective strategy for preserving a healthy diet, controlling weight, and promoting overall wellbeing. People can limit their calorie consumption, control their blood sugar levels, and achieve a better nutritional balance by controlling their portion sizes. Include doable tactics like making use of visual aids, reading food labels, using smaller dishes, estimating portions, organizing meals in advance, meditating, and getting help. Make portion control a permanent habit to reap the rewards of balanced eating and a healthy lifestyle. Keep in mind that altering your portion sizes can have a significant impact on your general wellbeing.

BUILDING BALANCED PLATE

A nutritious diet is built on a balanced plate, which gives your body the vital nutrients it needs to thrive. By comprehending the fundamentals of creating a balanced plate, you can make educated decisions about the foods you eat, support overall wellness, and encourage overall health. Let's examine the essential elements of a balanced plate, go through the advantages of this strategy, and offer helpful advice on how to put together balanced meals.

The common elements that make up a balanced plate are;

Lean protein: Each meal should contain a source of lean protein. Fish, poultry, lean meat, eggs, lentils, and plant-based substitutes like tofu or tempeh are examples of this. For the body to function properly and for muscles to grow and mend, one needs protein.

Whole Grains: Include whole grains in your meals, such as oats, brown rice, quinoa, whole wheat bread, and quinoa. Whole grains are a good source of fiber, vitamins, and minerals that provide you long-lasting energy and support your digestive system.

Fruits and veggies: Pile a variety of vibrant fruits and veggies onto half of your plate. They are stocked with vital nutrients including vitamins, minerals, and antioxidants that boost the immune system and lower the risk of chronic illnesses.

Healthy Fats: Incorporate healthy fat sources into your diet, such as avocados, nuts, seeds, olive oil, or fatty fish like salmon. Energy-giving, beneficial to brain health, and helping the body absorb fat-soluble vitamins are all functions of healthy fats.

Dairy or Dairy Alternatives: Include dairy foods like milk, yogurt, or cheese in your meals if you can tolerate them. Choose fortified plant-based substitutes like almond or soy milk if your diet is dairy-free.

A balanced plate guarantees that you get a variety of important nutrients, such as vitamins, minerals, protein, fiber, and healthy fats. This lowers the possibility of vitamin deficiency while promoting general health and supporting physical functioning.

So also, a balanced release of energy is provided throughout the day by the mix of protein, whole grains, fruits, and vegetables. This promotes steady blood sugar levels, avoids energy slumps, and sustains both physical and mental endurance. A balanced plate encourages portion control and offers a gratifying variety of nutrients, which helps with weight management. It makes you feel satisfied and full, which lowers your risk of overeating or reaching for junk food.

Chronic diseases including heart disease, diabetes, and some cancers are linked to a lower chance of eating a balanced plate full of fruits, vegetables, healthy grains, and lean proteins. An immune system that is strong and general wellbeing are supported by the richness of minerals and antioxidants.

A quick and easy way to eat healthily is to create a balanced plate. You can make sure you're giving your body the nutrients it needs for optimal operation by consuming protein, whole grains, fruits, vegetables, healthy fats, and dairy or dairy substitutes. Accept portion management, value whole foods, and attentive meal planning. Remember that a balanced plate is the basis for a healthy, vigorous existence in addition to being aesthetically pleasing. Start assembling a balanced plate right away to start reaping the rewards of a healthy diet.

Effective diabetes management requires portion control and creating a balanced plate, they help with diabetes management in the following ways

•Blood Sugar Management: Portion control is essential for blood sugar management. You can regulate your carbohydrate intake, which directly affects blood glucose levels, by managing the amount of food you eat at each meal. Consuming the right amount of food on a regular basis helps minimize blood sugar increases and improves glucose control.

•Carbohydrate Management: Since carbohydrates have the greatest influence on blood sugar levels, managing diabetes frequently entails monitoring and restricting carbohydrate intake. Including the right amount of carbohydrates on your plate, together with protein, healthy fats, and fiber-rich fruits and vegetables, guarantees that you are eating a balanced diet. This well-rounded strategy improves diabetes management by assisting in the maintenance of stable blood sugar levels.

•Weight management: For those with diabetes, weight management is crucial. Portion control and creating a balanced plate can help. You can create a calorie balance that supports healthy weight management or, if necessary, weight loss by regulating portion sizes and consuming a balanced mix of nutrients. Keeping a healthy weight helps optimize blood sugar regulation, improve insulin sensitivity, and lower the risk of complications from diabetes.

•Nutritional Intake: To manage diabetes, it's important to consume the right nutrients while keeping a close eye on your carbohydrate intake. By creating a balanced plate, you can make sure that you get a variety of nutrients from a variety of food sources, such as vitamins, minerals, fiber, and healthy fats. This balanced approach encourages optimal physical functions, improves general health, and helps avoid dietary deficits.

•Long-Lasting Energy: A balanced plate with reasonable portion sizes gives you long-lasting energy all day long. Proteins, good fats, and fiber slow down digestion and cause a steady release of glucose into the circulation when consumed with carbohydrates. This contributes to general wellbeing by reducing blood sugar rises and offering a consistent supply of energy, preventing energy crashes.

•Better Medication Management: For people with diabetes, portion control and creating balanced meals can also help with medication management. You can better coordinate your medication dosages to maximize blood sugar control by maintaining constant portion sizes and consuming carbohydrates equally throughout the day.

Overall, portion control and assembling a balanced plate are essential to effectively controlling diabetes. They support medication management, promote weight management, ensure nutrient adequacy, provide sustained energy, and help control blood sugar levels and carbohydrate intake. Together with advice from medical professionals, including these habits into your everyday routine can help you better manage your diabetes and live a healthier life.

CHAPTER 4

IDEAL MEAL PLAN

A diabetes diet must place a strong emphasis on the correct foods. You may manage blood sugar levels, maintain a healthy weight, and promote overall wellbeing by putting an emphasis on nutrient-dense foods. In a diabetes diet, it's important to focus the following foods:

Non-Starchy veggies: Non-starchy veggies are a great option for treating diabetes because they are high in fiber and low in carbs. Include a range of foods, such as bell peppers, cucumbers, zucchini, cauliflower, broccoli, and leafy greens (spinach, kale). While being low in calories, these vegetables offer important vitamins, minerals, and antioxidants.

Whole Grains: To guarantee a consistent release of glucose into the bloodstream, choose whole grains over refined grains. Whole grains are high in fiber and include healthy nutrients, such as quinoa, brown rice, oats, whole wheat bread, and whole wheat pasta. They can encourage satiety and help control blood sugar levels.

Lean Proteins: To reduce your intake of saturated fat, choose lean sources of protein. Lean cuts of beef or pork, skinless chicken, fish (such as salmon, trout, and tuna), tofu, tempeh, and legumes (beans, lentils, and chickpeas) are all good choices. Protein aids in satiety, muscular preservation, and blood sugar regulation.

Healthy Fats: Make sure your diabetes diet contains sources of healthy fats. Select foods high in monounsaturated and polyunsaturated fats, such as avocados, almonds, walnuts, chia seeds, flax seeds, and olive oil. These fats can enhance heart health, lower inflammation, and increase insulin sensitivity.

Fatty Fish: Omega-3 fatty acids, which are abundant in fatty fish like salmon, mackerel, sardines, and trout, have been demonstrated to provide a number of health advantages. Omega-3 fatty acids can lower inflammation, strengthen the heart, and promote brain health. At least two portions of fatty fish each week are recommended.

Low-Fat Dairy or Dairy Alternatives: If you can consume dairy products, go for low-fat varieties like skim milk, plain yogurt, or cottage cheese. These offer protein, calcium, and vitamin D. Choose fortified substitutes such unsweetened almond milk or soy milk if you maintain a dairy-free diet.

Berries: Berries, such as strawberries, blueberries, raspberries, and blackberries, are high in fiber and antioxidants while being low in sugar. While offering vital nutrients and aiding in overall blood sugar control, they can fulfill your sweet taste.

Nuts and Seeds: Nuts and seeds make great snack foods for those with diabetes. They offer fiber, good fats, and a range of vitamins and minerals. Great options include walnuts, chia seeds, flaxseeds, and pumpkin seeds.

Legumes: Legumes are rich in fiber, protein, and complex carbs. This group of foods includes beans, lentils, and chickpeas. They have a low glycemic index, which indicates that they barely affect blood sugar levels. Legumes can help regulate appetite and also contribute to a feeling of fullness.

Herbs and spices: Use herbs and spices to flavor your food without using additional salt or sugar. Cinnamon, turmeric, ginger, garlic, and oregano are a few examples of foods that may have extra health advantages in addition to decreasing blood sugar levels.

Keep in mind that unique dietary suggestions may change depending on personal health objectives and medical advice. A diabetes diet plan tailored to your individual requirements and tastes should be developed in collaboration with a qualified dietitian or other healthcare expert.

It's crucial to be aware of foods that can adversely affect blood sugar management when treating diabetes. While moderation is important, some meals are best avoided or limited in order to support overall health and maintain stable blood sugar levels. The following foods should be avoided when following a diabetes diet:

Sugary Beverages: Sugar-sweetened drinks with little to no nutritional value include soda, fruit juices, sweetened teas, and energy drinks. They are heavy in added sugars. These beverages can lead to weight gain and produce sharp spikes in blood sugar levels. It's preferable to choose beverages with no added sugars, including water, unsweetened tea, or flavored water.

Refined Grains: The fiber and nutrients have been removed from foods made from refined grains, including white bread, white rice, and processed cereals. These carbs breakdown fast, which might result in abrupt spikes in blood sugar levels. As an alternative, pick products made with whole grains including whole wheat, quinoa, brown rice, bread, and cereal.

Desserts and Sweets: Consume sugary foods like sweets, candies, pastries, cookies, cakes, and other desserts in moderation. These foods have a lot of calories, bad fats, and added sugars. When you're in the mood for something sweet, choose more nutritious options like fresh fruit, sugar-free treats, or small servings of dark chocolate that has at least 70% cocoa.

Processed Snack Foods: Packaged snacks like chips, crackers, and pretzels frequently have high levels of sodium, refined carbs, and harmful fats. These snacks have little nutritional value and can cause blood sugar to surge. Pick something healthier like nuts, seeds, fresh fruit, or homemade snacks prepared from whole foods.

High-Fat Meats: Avoid consuming excessive amounts of high-fat meats like bacon, sausage, hot dogs, and fatty cuts of beef, as well as full-fat dairy products. These meals include significant amounts of saturated fats, which raise the risk of heart disease and impair insulin sensitivity. Select skinless poultry, skinless fish, and plant-based protein sources as your protein sources of choice.

Trans Fats: Trans fats, which are present in many processed and fried meals, can raise the risk of inflammation and heart disease. Limit or stay away from items like margarine, fried foods, commercial baked products, and several packaged snacks that contain hydrogenated or partially hydrogenated oils.

Limit your consumption of items high in sodium, such as processed meats, canned soups, fast meals, and salty snacks. High salt intake raises the risk of cardiovascular problems and raises blood pressure. Instead, use low-sodium options and season food with herbs, spices, and other ingredients.

Sweetened Condiments and Sauces: Watch out for sauces and condiments with added sugars, like ketchup, barbecue sauce, and sweetened salad dressings. Choose options that are low in sugar or sugar-free, or think about creating your own healthy substitutes using natural sweeteners or vinegar-based dressings.

Alcohol: Some people with diabetes may be able to consume moderate amounts of alcohol, but it's crucial to talk to your doctor beforehand. Both alcohol and several diabetic treatments can reduce blood sugar levels. If you decide to drink, do so sparingly and think about selecting beverages like light beer, dry wine, or spirits blended with sugar-free mixers.

Fat and protein are crucial for managing diabetes, I mean really significant. Let's check out how protein helps in managing diabetes

Blood Sugar Control: Compared to carbs, protein has less effect on blood sugar levels. When combined with carbohydrates, protein can help slow down the release of glucose into the bloodstream, causing blood sugar levels to rise more gradually. This can help to prevent post-meal increases and maintain steady blood sugar levels.

Satiety and Weight Management: Foods high in protein are believed to increase satiety and a sensation of fullness. Including protein in your meals and snacks can help you manage your weight by reducing hunger and preventing overeating. For those with diabetes, maintaining a healthy weight is crucial since it helps enhance insulin sensitivity and overall blood sugar control.

Muscle Growth and Repair: Protein is essential for the growth, repair, and maintenance of muscles. Diabetes management requires regular exercise, and healthy protein consumption promotes the maintenance and repair of muscles. For those who practice resistance or strength training, this is very crucial.

Glucagon Regulation: Protein stimulates the hormone glucagon, which helps control blood sugar levels, from being released into the body. When blood sugar levels are low, glucagon promotes the breakdown of liver-stored glycogen and the release of glucose into the bloodstream in opposition to insulin. By doing this, hypoglycemia—or low blood sugar—is avoided.

Nutrient Density: Protein-rich foods frequently contain a variety of important vitamins, minerals, and amino acids, making them nutrient-dense diets. Lean sources of protein can help you make sure you get the essential nutrients required for general health and wellbeing.

Just like protein, fats also plays important roles in managing diabetes, roles like;

Blood Sugar Regulation: When ingested with carbs, healthy fats can help slow down the absorption of glucose into the bloodstream and have no effect on blood sugar levels. This may help improve blood sugar regulation and lessen the chance of blood sugar spikes.

Satiety and appetite control: Fats have more calories per gram than carbohydrates or protein and make you feel satiated and full after eating. Healthy fats can support portion control, appetite control, and preventing overeating by being included in your meals.

Insulin Sensitivity: Getting enough of the mono- and polyunsaturated fats, which are present in foods like avocados, nuts, seeds, and olive oil, might enhance insulin sensitivity. Consequently, cells become more receptive to insulin, enhancing glucose utilization and blood sugar regulation.

Heart Health: Diabetes is linked to a higher risk of developing heart disease. Omega-3 fatty acids, which are present in fatty fish like salmon and can help reduce inflammation and triglyceride levels, are particularly beneficial for heart health. For the management of cardiovascular risks associated with diabetes, choosing healthy fat sources over saturated and trans fats is crucial.

Nutrient Absorption: Some vitamins and minerals are fat-soluble, which means that they need fat for the body to absorb them effectively. Your body will absorb these necessary nutrients more effectively if you include healthy fats in your meals, which will improve your general health.

While protein and good fats are useful, it's crucial to remember that moderation and quantity control are essential.

CHAPTER 5

RECIPES

BREAKFAST RECIPES

Recipe 1

Veggie Omelette

For this recipe, you will need;

- 2 eggs

- ¼ cup diced bell peppers

- ¼ cup chopped spinach

- ¼ cup diced tomatoes

- 1 tablespoon chopped onions

- Salt and pepper to taste

Instructions

1. Whisk the eggs in a bowl and season with salt and pepper.

2. Heat a non-stick pan over medium heat and lightly coat with cooking spray.

3. Add the bell peppers, spinach, tomatoes, and onions to the pan and sauté for a few minutes until softened.

4. Pour the beaten eggs over the vegetables and cook until the eggs are set.

5. Flip the omelette and cook for another minute.

6. Serve hot with a side of whole grain toast or a small portion of cooked quinoa.

Recipe 2: Greek Yogurt Parfait:

For this recipe, you will need;

- ½ cup plain Greek yogurt

- ¼ cup mixed berries (such as blueberries, raspberries, or strawberries)

- 1 tablespoon chopped nuts (almonds, walnuts, or pistachios)

- 1 teaspoon honey (optional)

Instructions

1. In a glass or bowl, layer the Greek yogurt, mixed berries, and chopped nuts.

2. Drizzle with honey, if desired, for added sweetness.

3. Enjoy as is or refrigerate overnight for a ready-to-eat breakfast option.

Recipe 3: Overnight Chia Pudding

For this recipe, you will need;

- 2 tablespoons chia seeds

- ½ cup unsweetened almond milk or any milk of choice

- ¼ teaspoon vanilla extract

- 1 tablespoon chopped nuts or seeds

- Fresh berries for topping

Instructions:

1. In a jar or container, combine chia seeds, almond milk, and vanilla extract.

2. Stir well to evenly distribute the chia seeds.

3. Cover and refrigerate overnight or for at least 4 hours.

4. Stir the mixture again before serving.

5. Top with chopped nuts or seeds and fresh berries.

Recipe 4: Whole Grain Toast with Avocado and Egg

For this recipe, you will need;

- 1 slice of whole grain bread

- ¼ ripe avocado, mashed

- 1 boiled egg, sliced

- Salt and pepper to taste

Instructions:

1. Toast the whole grain bread to your desired level of crispness.

2. Spread the mashed avocado on the toasted bread.

3. Place the sliced boiled egg on top.

4. Season with salt and pepper.

5. Serve with a side of fresh fruit or a small serving of low-fat cottage cheese.

Recipe 5: Berry Protein Smoothie

For this recipe, you will need;

- ½ cup unsweetened almond milk or any milk of choice

- ½ cup plain Greek yogurt

- ½ cup mixed berries (such as blueberries, raspberries, or strawberries)

- 1 tablespoon almond butter or peanut butter

- 1 tablespoon chia seeds (optional)

- Ice cubes (optional)

Instructions:

1. Place all the ingredients in a blender.

2. Blend until smooth and creamy.

3. If desired, add ice cubes for a chilled texture.

4. Pour into a glass and enjoy.

Recipe 6: Quinoa Breakfast Bowl:

For this recipe, you will need;

- ½ cup cooked quinoa

- ¼ cup sliced almonds or other nuts/seeds

- ¼ cup diced fresh fruit (such as apples, berries, or banana)

- 1 tablespoon unsweetened shredded coconut

- Cinnamon powder to taste

Instructions:

1. In a bowl, combine cooked quinoa, sliced almonds, diced fruit, shredded coconut, and a sprinkle of cinnamon Powder.
2. Mix well and adjust sweetness with a natural sweetener like stevia or a drizzle of honey, if desired. Serve and enjoy

Recipe 7: Vegetable Breakfast Burrito:

For this recipe, you will need;

- 1 whole wheat tortilla

- 2 eggs, scrambled

- ¼ cup diced bell peppers

- ¼ cup diced onions

- ¼ cup chopped spinach

- ¼ cup salsa (optional)

Instructions:

1. Heat a non-stick pan over medium heat and lightly coat with cooking spray.

2. Add the bell peppers, onions, and spinach to the pan and sauté until softened.

3. Add the scrambled eggs and cook until they are fully cooked through.

4. Warm the whole wheat tortilla in a separate pan or microwave.

5. Place the vegetable and egg mixture onto the tortilla, and add salsa if desired.

6. Roll up the tortilla to form a burrito and enjoy.

Recipe 8: Cottage Cheese and Fruit Bowl:

For this recipe, you will need;

- ½ cup low-fat cottage cheese

- ¼ cup diced fresh fruit (such as pineapple, mango, or melon)

- 1 tablespoon chopped nuts or seeds (optional)

- Cinnamon powder to taste

Instructions:

1. In a bowl, combine low-fat cottage cheese, diced fresh fruit, chopped nuts or seeds, and a sprinkle of cinnamon powder.

2. Mix well and enjoy as is or refrigerate for a refreshing breakfast option.

Recipe 9: Smoked Salmon Wrap:

For this recipe, you will need;

- 1 whole grain wrap or tortilla

- 2 ounces smoked salmon

- 2 tablespoons cream cheese (low-fat or light)

- Thinly sliced cucumber and red onion

Instructions:

1. Spread the cream cheese evenly over the whole grain wrap or tortilla.

2. Place the smoked salmon, cucumber slices, and red onion on top.

3. Roll up the wrap tightly.

4. Slice it into smaller sections if desired.

5. Serve with a side salad or vegetable sticks.

Recipe 10: Vegetable Frittata Muffins:

For this recipe, you will need;

- 4 large eggs

- ¼ cup diced bell peppers

- ¼ cup diced onions

- ¼ cup chopped spinach

- Salt and pepper to taste

Instructions:

1. Preheat the oven to 350°F (175°C) and grease a muffin tin.

2. In a bowl, whisk the eggs and season with salt and pepper.

3. Stir in the diced bell peppers, onions, and chopped spinach.

4. Pour the mixture evenly into the greased muffin tin.

5. Bake for about 15-20 minutes or until the frittata muffins are set and slightly golden.

6. Allow them to cool slightly before removing them from the tin.

7. Serve as a grab-and-go breakfast option or enjoy with a side salad.

LUNCH AND DINNER RECIPES

Recipe 1: Grilled Chicken with Roasted Vegetables

For this recipe, you will need;

- 4 ounces boneless, skinless chicken breast

- Assorted vegetables (such as bell peppers, zucchini, and broccoli)

- 1 tablespoon olive oil

- Garlic powder, salt, and pepper to taste

Instructions:

1. Preheat the grill to medium heat.

2. Season the chicken breast with garlic powder, salt, and pepper.

3. Grill the chicken for about 6-8 minutes per side or until cooked through.

4. Meanwhile, toss the assorted vegetables with olive oil, garlic powder, salt, and pepper.

5. Roast the vegetables in the oven at 400°F (200°C) for about 20 minutes or until tender.

6. Serve the grilled chicken with roasted vegetables for a balanced and satisfying meal.

Recipe 2: Baked Salmon with Quinoa and Steamed Broccoli

For this recipe, you will need;

- 4 ounces salmon fillet

- ½ cup cooked quinoa

- Steamed broccoli florets

- Lemon juice

- Dill, salt, and pepper to taste

Instructions:

1. Preheat the oven to 375°F (190°C).

2. Place the salmon fillet on a baking sheet lined with parchment paper.

3. Season the salmon with lemon juice, dill, salt, and pepper.

4. Bake for about 15-20 minutes or until the salmon is cooked through.

5. Serve the baked salmon with a side of cooked quinoa and steamed broccoli.

Recipe 3: Turkey and Vegetable Stir-Fry

For this recipe, you will need;

- 4 ounces ground turkey

- Assorted stir-fry vegetables (such as bell peppers, snap peas, carrots, and mushrooms)

- 1 tablespoon low-sodium soy sauce

- 1 teaspoon sesame oil

- Garlic powder, ginger powder, salt, and pepper to taste

Instructions:

1. In a non-stick skillet, cook the ground turkey until browned and cooked through.

2. Add the stir-fry vegetables to the skillet and sauté until tender.

3. Season with garlic powder, ginger powder, salt, and pepper.

4. Stir in the low-sodium soy sauce and sesame oil.

5. Cook for an additional minute or until the flavors are well combined.

6. Serve the turkey and vegetable stir-fry over a bed of cauliflower rice or brown rice.

Recipe 4: Chickpea Salad

For this recipe, you will need;

- 1 cup cooked chickpeas

- Chopped vegetables (such as cucumber, cherry tomatoes, red onion, and bell peppers)

- Chopped fresh herbs (such as parsley or cilantro)

- Juice of 1 lemon

- 1 tablespoon olive oil

- Salt and pepper to taste

Instructions:

1. In a bowl, combine the cooked chickpeas, chopped vegetables, and fresh herbs.

2. Drizzle with lemon juice and olive oil.

3. Season with salt and pepper.

4. Toss well to combine all the ingredients.

5. Let the flavors marinate for a few minutes before serving.

6. Enjoy the chickpea salad as a light and refreshing lunch option.

Recipe 5: Quinoa Stuffed Bell Peppers

For this recipe, you will need;

- 2 large bell peppers

- 1 cup cooked quinoa

- Ground turkey or lean ground beef (optional)

- Chopped vegetables (such as onions, zucchini, and carrots)

- ¼ cup tomato sauce (no added sugar)

- Garlic powder, cumin, salt, and pepper to taste

Instructions:

1. Preheat the oven to 375°F (190°C).

2. Cut the tops off the bell peppers and remove the seeds and membranes.

3. In a skillet, cook the ground turkey or lean ground beef (if using) until browned.

4. Add the chopped vegetables to the skillet and sauté until tender.

5. Stir in the cooked quinoa, tomato sauce, and seasonings.

6. Stuff the bell peppers with the quinoa and meat mixture.

7. Place the stuffed bell peppers in a baking dish and cover with foil.

8. Bake for about 30-35 minutes or until the bell peppers are tender.

9. Remove the foil and bake for an additional 5 minutes to lightly brown the tops.

10. Serve the quinoa stuffed bell peppers as a hearty and nutritious dinner option.

Recipe 6: Lentil Soup

For this recipe, you will need;

- 1 cup cooked lentils

- Chopped vegetables (such as onions, carrots, celery, and tomatoes)

- Low-sodium vegetable broth

- Garlic powder, cumin, paprika, salt, and pepper to taste

Instructions:

1. In a large pot, sauté the chopped vegetables until they begin to soften.

2. Add the cooked lentils and enough vegetable broth to cover the ingredients.

3. Season with garlic powder, cumin, paprika, salt, and pepper.

4. Bring the soup to a boil, then reduce the heat and simmer for about 20-25 minutes.

5. Adjust the seasonings if needed.

6. Serve the lentil soup with a side of whole grain bread or a small green salad.

Recipe 7: Grilled Shrimp and Vegetable Skewers

For this recipe, you will need;

- 4 ounces shrimp, peeled and deveined

- Assorted vegetables (such as cherry tomatoes, bell peppers, zucchini, and mushrooms)

- 1 tablespoon olive oil

- Lemon juice

- Garlic powder, dried herbs, salt, and pepper to taste

Instructions:

1. Preheat the grill to medium heat.

2. In a bowl, toss the shrimp and vegetables with olive oil, lemon juice, garlic powder, dried herbs, salt, and pepper.

3. Thread the shrimp and vegetables onto skewers.

4. Grill the skewers for about 2-3 minutes per side or until the shrimp are pink and cooked through.

5. Serve the grilled shrimp and vegetable skewers with a side of quinoa or whole grain couscous.

Recipe 8: Baked Chicken Breast with Sweet Potato and Steamed Green Beans

For this recipe, you will need;

- 4 ounces chicken breast

- 1 small sweet potato, diced

- Steamed green beans

- Olive oil

- Garlic powder, paprika, salt, and pepper to taste

Instructions:

1. Preheat the oven to 375°F (190°C).

2. Place the chicken breast on a baking sheet lined with parchment paper.

3. Drizzle with olive oil and season with garlic powder, paprika, salt, and pepper.

4. Bake for about 20-25 minutes or until the chicken is cooked through.

5. Meanwhile, toss the diced sweet potato with olive oil, garlic powder, paprika, salt, and pepper.

6. Roast the sweet potato in the oven at 375°F (190°C) for about 20-25 minutes or until tender.

7. Serve the baked chicken breast with roasted sweet potato and steamed green beans.

Recipe 9: Spinach and Feta Stuffed Chicken Breast:

For this recipe, you will need;

- 4 ounces chicken breast

- ¼ cup cooked spinach, squeezed to remove excess moisture

- 1 tablespoon crumbled feta cheese

- Garlic powder, dried herbs, salt, and pepper to taste

Instructions:

1. Preheat the oven to 375°F (190°C).

2. Cut a slit in the side of the chicken breast to create a pocket for stuffing.

3. In a small bowl, mix together the cooked spinach, feta cheese, garlic powder, dried herbs, salt, and pepper.

4. Stuff the mixture into the pocket of the chicken breast.

5. Place the stuffed chicken breast on a baking sheet lined with parchment paper.

6. Bake for about 25-30 minutes or until the chicken is cooked through.

7. Serve the spinach and feta stuffed chicken breast with a side of roasted vegetables or a green salad.

Recipe 10: Vegetable Stir-Fry with Tofu

For this recipe, you will need;

- 4 ounces tofu, drained and cubed

- Assorted stir-fry vegetables (such as broccoli, snap peas, carrots, and mushrooms)

- Low-sodium soy sauce

- Garlic powder, ginger powder, salt, and pepper to taste

Instructions

1. In a non-stick skillet, cook the tofu until lightly browned on all sides.

2. Remove the tofu from the skillet and set aside.

3. Add the stir-fry vegetables to the skillet and sauté until tender.

4. Return the tofu to the skillet and season with garlic powder, ginger powder, salt, and pepper.

5. Drizzle with low-sodium soy sauce and cook for an additional minute.

6. Serve the vegetable stir-fry with tofu over a bed of brown rice or quinoa.

SNACKS AND DESSERT

Recipe 1: Greek Yogurt Parfait

For this recipe, you will need;

- ½ cup plain Greek yogurt

- ¼ cup fresh berries (such as strawberries, blueberries, or raspberries)

- 1 tablespoon chopped nuts or seeds (such as almonds or chia seeds)

- Cinnamon powder to taste

Instructions:

1. In a glass or bowl, layer the Greek yogurt, fresh berries, and chopped nuts or seeds.

2. Sprinkle with cinnamon powder.

3. Repeat the layers if desired.

4. Enjoy this protein-rich and satisfying snack.

Recipe 2: Veggie Sticks with Hummus

For this recipe, you will need;

- Assorted vegetable sticks (such as carrot sticks, cucumber slices, and bell pepper strips)

- 2 tablespoons hummus (choose a low-fat or homemade version)

Instructions:

1. Wash and cut the vegetables into sticks or slices.

2. Serve the vegetable sticks with hummus as a crunchy and nutritious snack.

Recipe 3: Apple Slices with Peanut Butter:

For this recipe, you will need;

- 1 medium apple, sliced

- 1 tablespoon natural peanut butter (without added sugar)

Instructions:

1. Slice the apple into thin rounds or wedges.

2. Spread each slice with a thin layer of peanut butter.

3. Enjoy the combination of sweet and savory flavors.

Recipe 4: Hard-Boiled Eggs:

You will need;

-2 hard-boiled eggs

Instructions:

1. Prepare the hard-boiled eggs by boiling them until cooked through.

2. Let them cool and enjoy as a protein-rich snack.

Recipe 5: Roasted Chickpeas

For this recipe, you will need;

- 1 can chickpeas, drained and rinsed

- 1 tablespoon olive oil

- Salt, pepper, and spices of choice (such as paprika, cumin, or chili powder)

Instructions:

1. Preheat the oven to 400°F (200°C) and line a baking sheet with parchment paper.

2. Pat dry the chickpeas with a clean towel.

3. In a bowl, toss the chickpeas with olive oil, salt, pepper, and desired spices.

4. Spread the chickpeas in a single layer on the baking sheet.

5. Roast in the oven for about 25-30 minutes or until crispy.

6. Allow them to cool before enjoying this crunchy and fiber-rich snack.

Recipe 6: Cottage Cheese with Berries:

For this recipe, you will need;

- ½ cup low-fat cottage cheese

- ¼ cup fresh berries (such as strawberries, blueberries, or raspberries)

- Cinnamon powder to taste

Instructions:

1. In a bowl, combine the low-fat cottage cheese and fresh berries.

2. Sprinkle with cinnamon powder for added flavor.

3. Enjoy this protein-packed snack.

Recipe 7: Cucumber and Tuna Bites

For this recipe, you will need;

- Cucumber slices

- 2 ounces canned tuna, drained

- Lemon juice

- Salt and pepper to taste

Instructions:

1. Place the cucumber slices on a plate or serving tray.

2. In a bowl, mix the drained tuna with lemon juice, salt, and pepper.

3. Top each cucumber slice with a small spoonful of the tuna mixture.

4. Enjoy this light and refreshing snack.

Recipe 8: Homemade Trail Mix:

For this recipe, you will need;

- ¼ cup unsalted nuts (such as almonds, walnuts, or cashews)

- ¼ cup unsalted seeds (such as pumpkin seeds or sunflower seeds)

- 2 tablespoons dried fruits (such as cranberries or apricots)

- 1 tablespoon dark chocolate chips (optional)

Instructions:

1. In a bowl, combine the unsalted nuts, seeds, dried fruits, and dark chocolate chips (if using).
2. Mix well and portion into small snack-sized bags for easy grab-and-go snacks.

Recipe 9: Baked Apple Chips

For this recipe, you will need;

- 1 medium apple, thinly sliced

- Cinnamon powder to taste

Instructions:

1. Preheat the oven to 200°F (95°C) and line a baking sheet with parchment paper.

2. Place the apple slices on the baking sheet in a single layer.

3. Sprinkle with cinnamon powder.

4. Bake in the oven for about 1.5-2 hours or until the apple slices are crisp.

5. Let them cool before enjoying these naturally sweet and crispy chips.

Recipe 10: Sugar-Free Chia Pudding

For this recipe, you will need;

- 2 tablespoons chia seeds

- 1 cup unsweetened almond milk (or any non-dairy milk of choice)

- Sugar substitute to taste (such as stevia or monk fruit)

Instructions:

1. In a bowl, mix the chia seeds and almond milk.

2. Add the sugar substitute and stir well.

3. Refrigerate for at least 2 hours or overnight to allow the chia seeds to absorb the liquid and create a pudding-like texture.

4. Serve chilled and top with fresh berries or chopped nuts if desired.

HOMEMADE DRINKS FOR YOU

Recipe 1: Green Smoothie:

For this recipe, you will need;

- 1 cup fresh spinach

- ½ medium cucumber

- ½ medium avocado

- ½ cup unsweetened almond milk (or any non-dairy milk of choice)

- Juice of ½ lemon

- Ice cubes (optional)

Instructions:

1. In a blender, combine the fresh spinach, cucumber, avocado, almond milk, and lemon juice.

2. Blend until smooth and creamy.

3. Add ice cubes if desired and blend again.

4. Serve chilled as a nutrient-packed green smoothie.

Recipe 2: Berry Blast Smoothie:

For this recipe, you will need;

- ½ cup fresh or frozen berries (such as strawberries, blueberries, or raspberries)

- ½ medium banana

- ½ cup plain Greek yogurt

- ½ cup unsweetened almond milk (or any non-dairy milk of choice)

- Ice cubes (optional)

Instructions:

1. In a blender, combine the berries, banana, Greek yogurt, and almond milk.

2. Blend until smooth and well combined.

3. Add ice cubes if desired and blend again.

4. Serve chilled as a delicious and fruity smoothie.

Recipe 3: Iced Herbal Tea

For this recipe, you will need;

- 2 herbal tea bags (such as chamomile, mint, or hibiscus)

- 2 cups boiling water

- Ice cubes

- Lemon or lime slices for garnish (optional)

Instructions:

1. Place the herbal tea bags in a large heatproof pitcher.

2. Pour the boiling water over the tea bags and let steep for 5-10 minutes.

3. Remove the tea bags and let the tea cool to room temperature.

4. Once cooled, refrigerate the tea until chilled.

5. Serve the iced herbal tea over ice cubes.

6. Garnish with lemon or lime slices if desired.

7. Enjoy this refreshing and caffeine-free beverage.

Recipe 4: Sparkling Water with Citrus:

For this recipe, you will need;

- 1 cup sparkling water

- Juice of ½ lemon or lime

- Slices of lemon or lime for garnish

- Stevia or other sugar substitute to taste (optional)

Instructions:

1. Fill a glass with sparkling water.

2. Squeeze the juice of half a lemon or lime into the glass.

3. Add a few slices of lemon or lime for extra flavor.

4. If desired, sweeten with stevia or any other sugar substitute.

5. Stir well and serve chilled.

6. This fizzy and tangy drink is a refreshing option.

Recipe 5: Cucumber and Mint Infused Water

For this recipe, you will need;

- ½ medium cucumber, sliced

- Fresh mint leaves

- Water

- Ice cubes

Instructions:

1. Place the cucumber slices and fresh mint leaves in a large pitcher.

2. Fill the pitcher with water.

3. Stir gently to combine the ingredients.

4. Refrigerate the infused water for at least 2 hours to allow the flavors to meld.

5. Serve chilled over ice cubes.

6. Enjoy this hydrating and flavorful infused water.

Feel free to adjust the recipes based on personal preferences and dietary restrictions. It's always a good idea to consult with a registered dietitian or healthcare professional for personalized advice. Enjoy these healthy, sumptuous and refreshing and diabetes-friendly homemade recipes.